The Daddy Haircut

written by

Nicole Cable Scoubes

with illustrations by Joel Cable

To my wonderful daughter Mia
who always made me feel beautiful,
and my sweet Macie who held me so tight.

I will be with you no matter
where you go or what you do.

I hope this book reminds you of
my love for both of you
always.

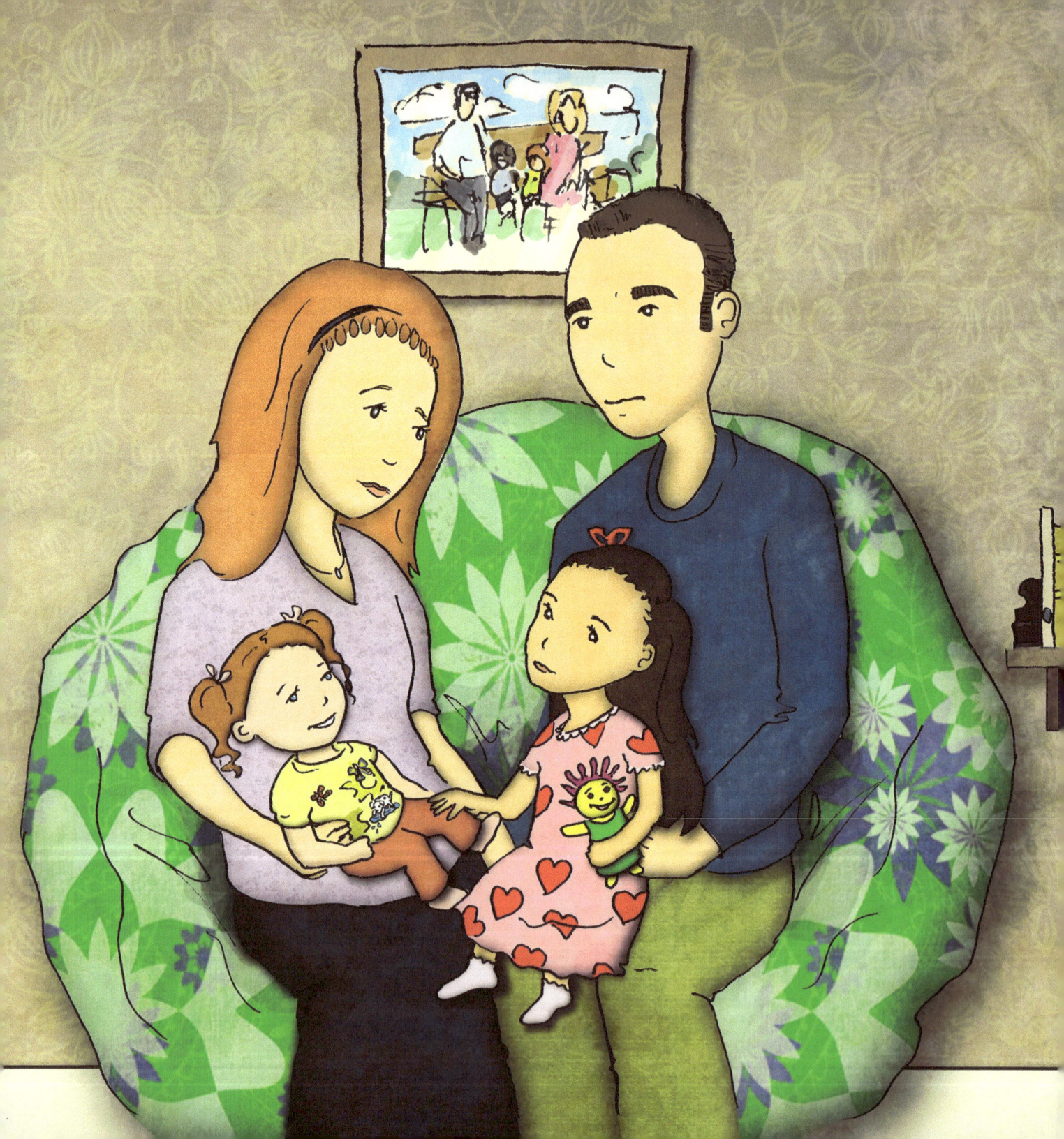

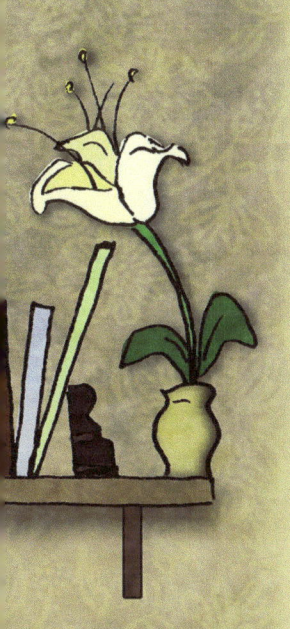

Mommy tells us
she has cancer,
and medicine will
make her better.

She says she will
have a 'daddy haircut',
and the doctors
are going to help her.

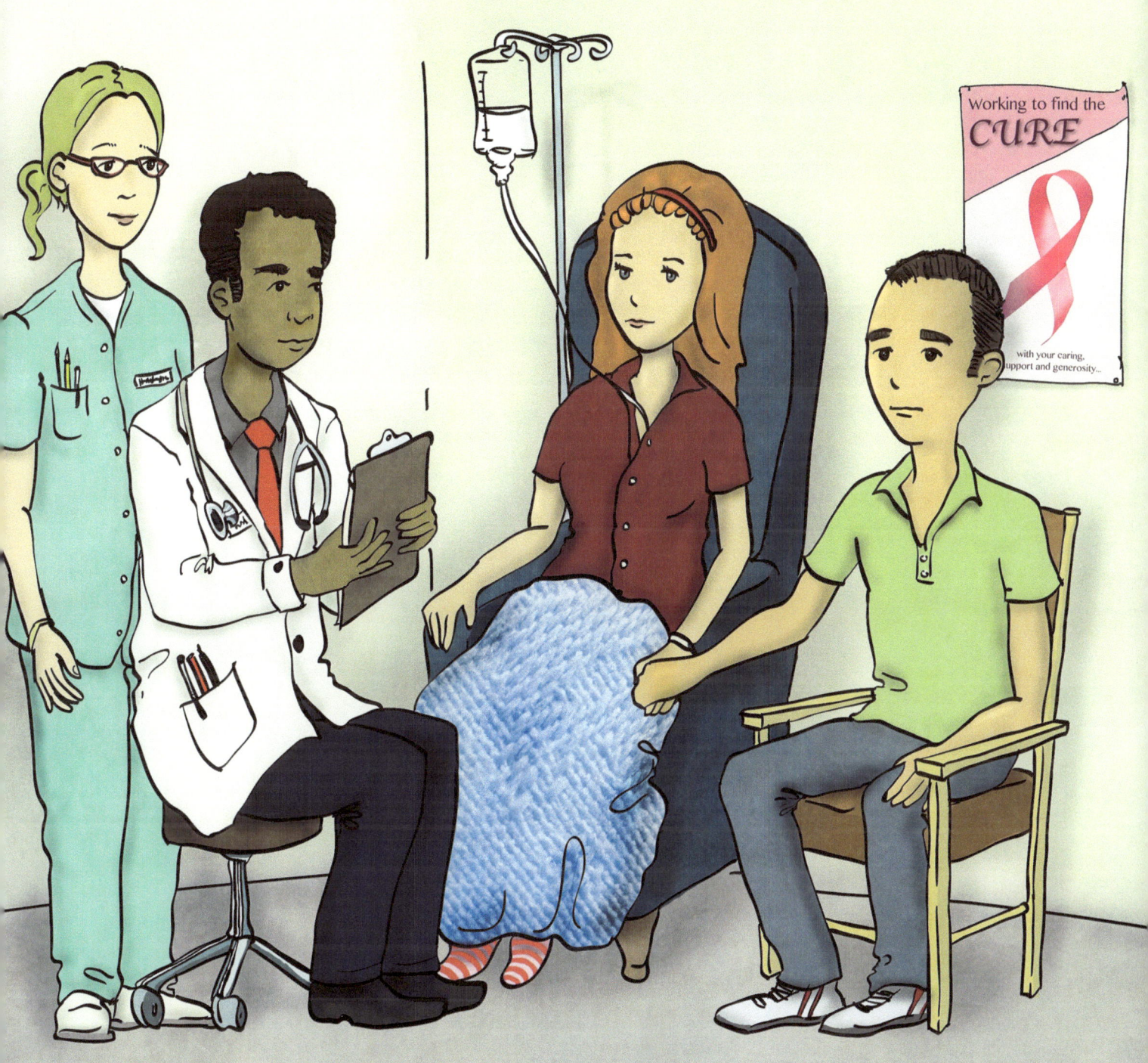

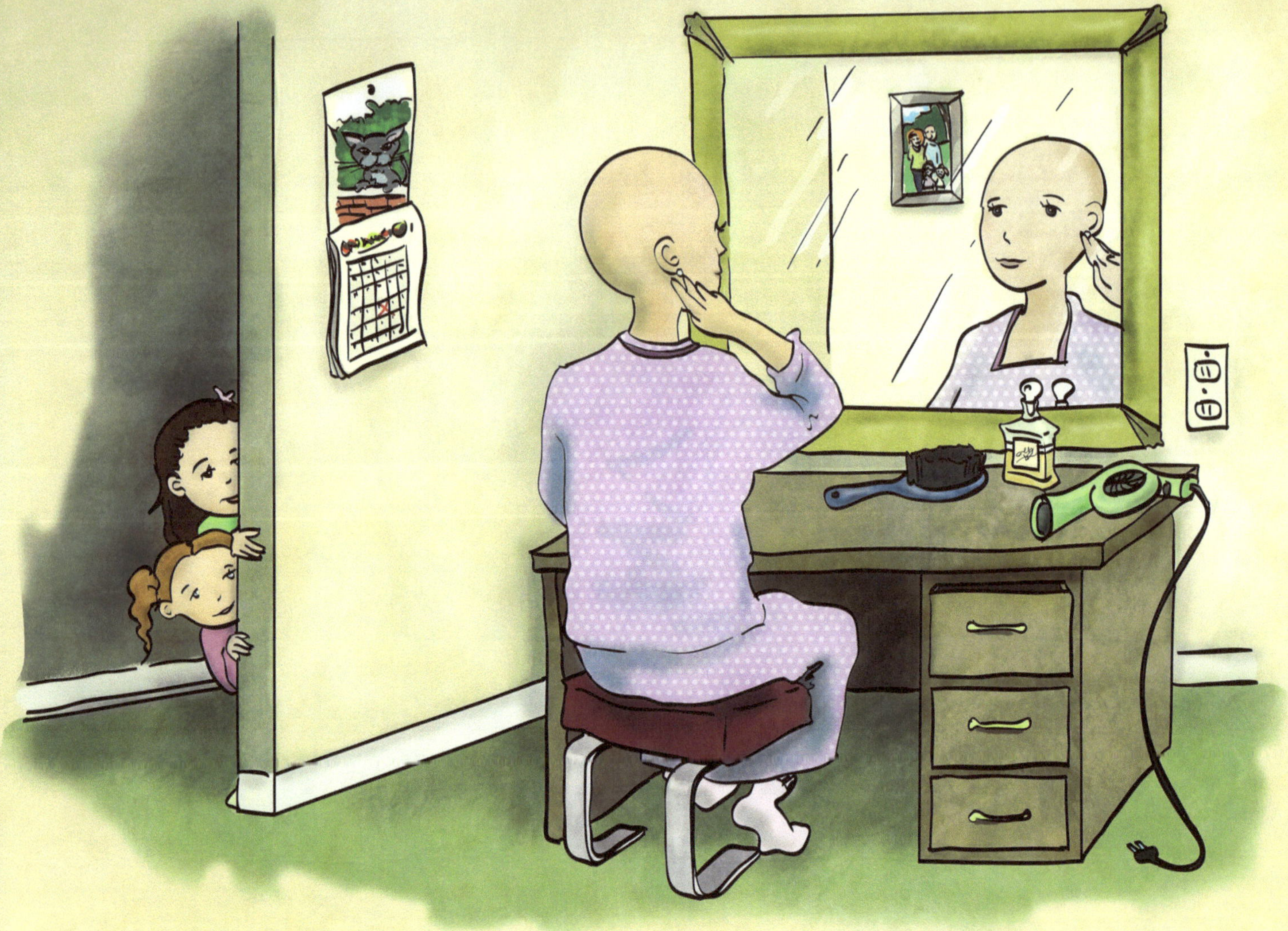

Mom and Dad say things will
change, more than just her looks.

Friends and neighbors bring us dinner so Dad won't have to cook!

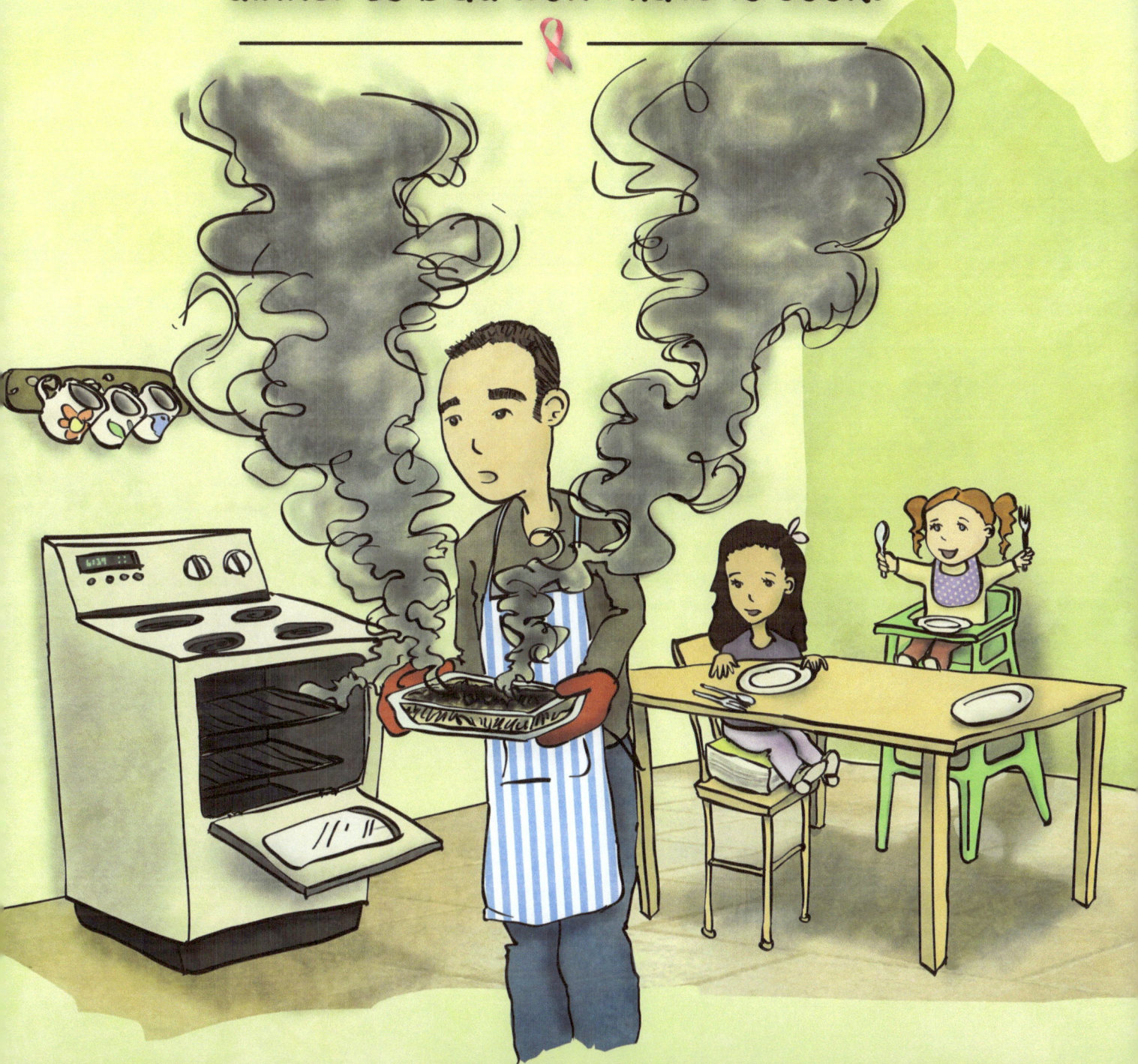

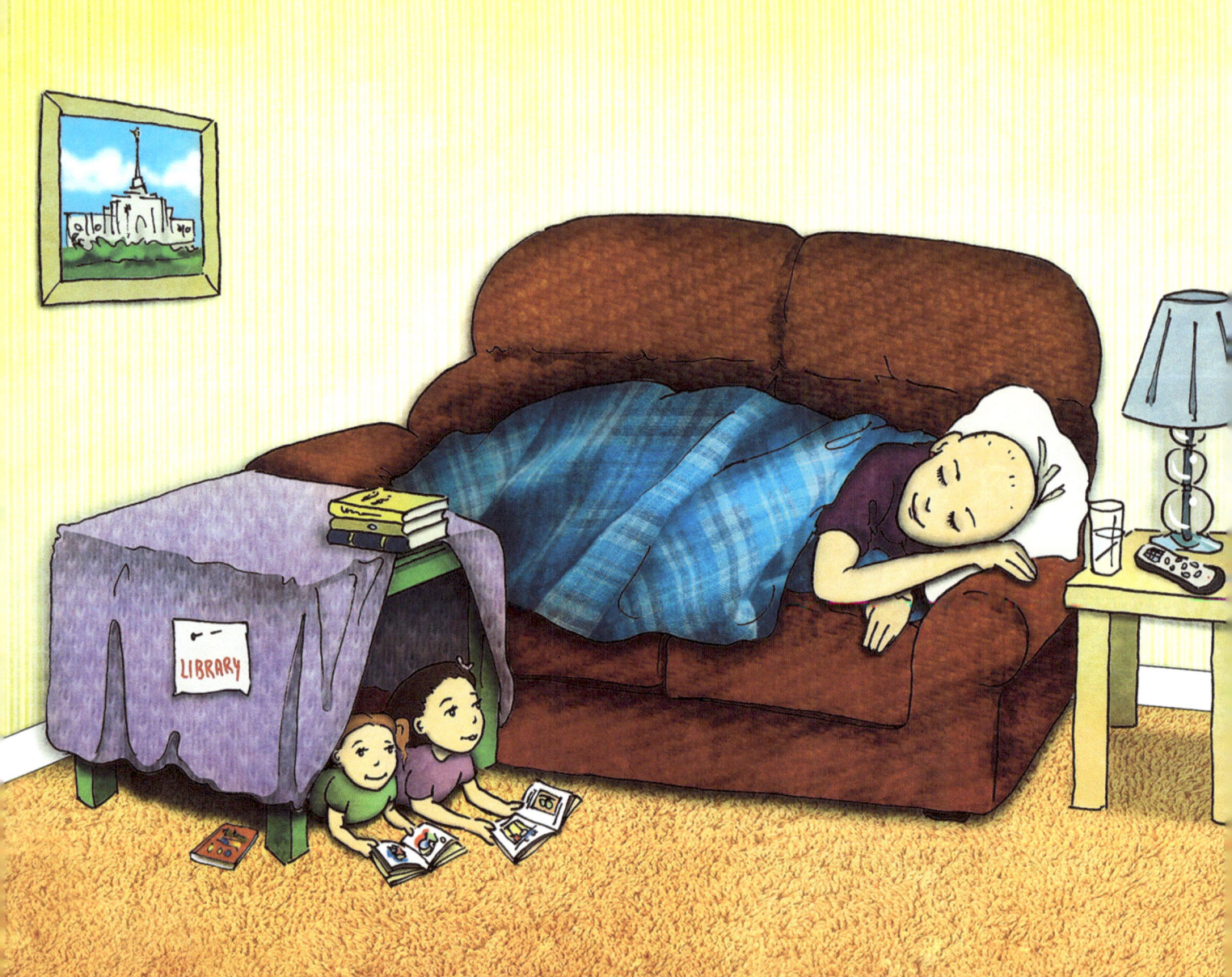

Mommy likes the couch a lot more than she did before.

We read our books and play pretend beside her on the floor.

——————— ✦ ———————

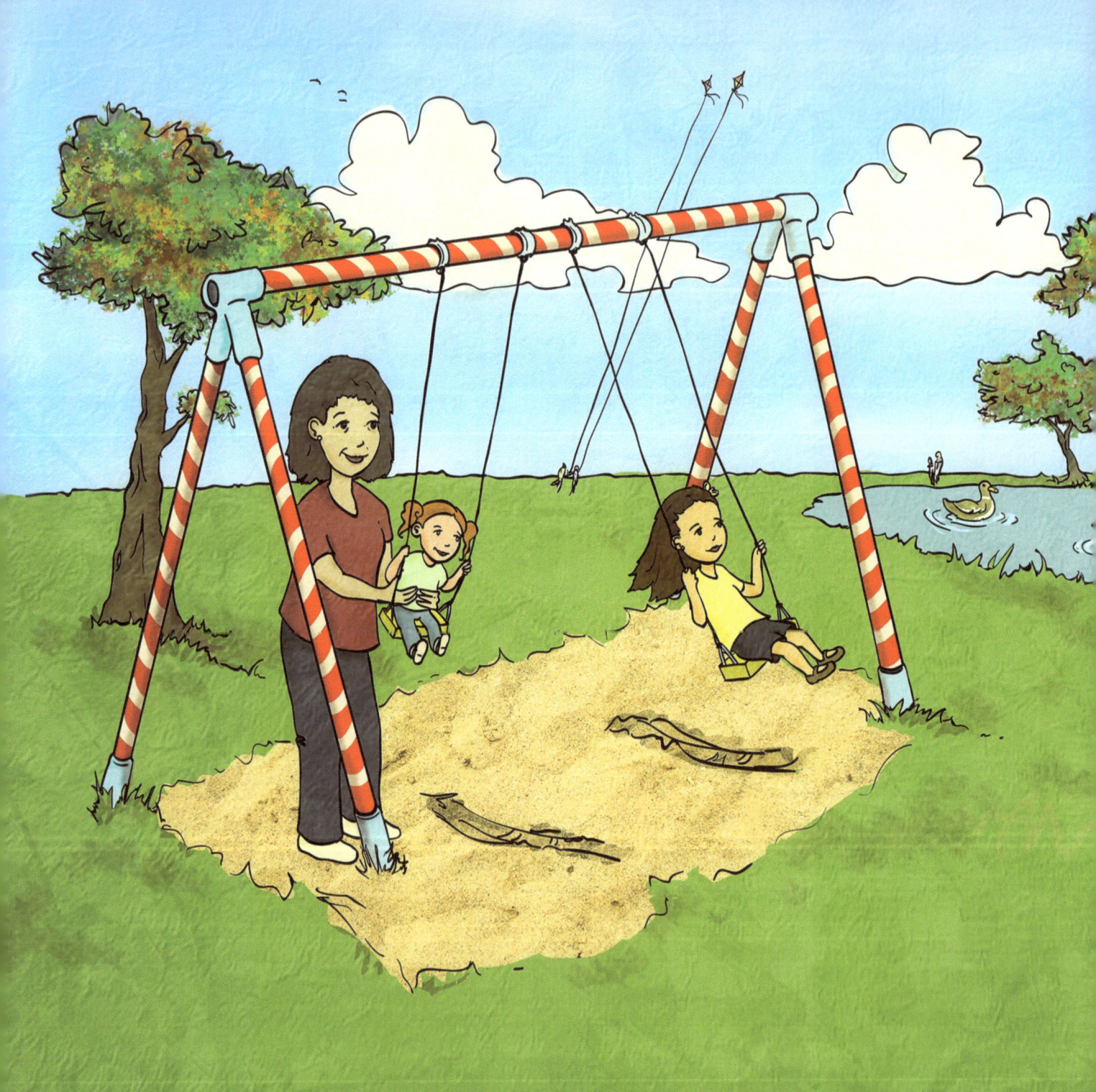

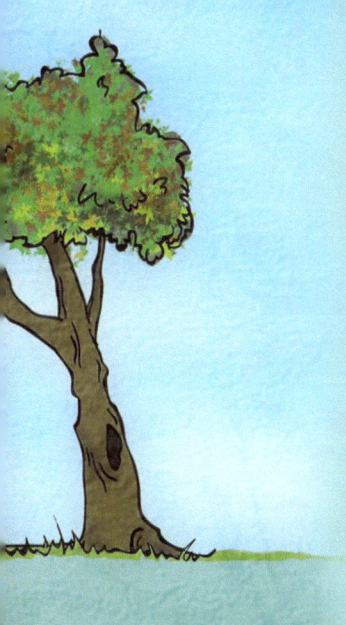

We have lots of fun
with Grandma every
single week.

Off to the park
and out to lunch so
Mom can get
some sleep!

——————— ———————

Mommy got so many
shapes and colors
of pretty hats.

She even got a few
nice wigs, but we use
those for laughs!

——————— 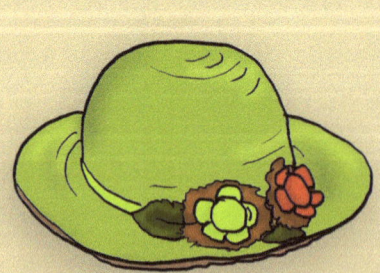 ———————

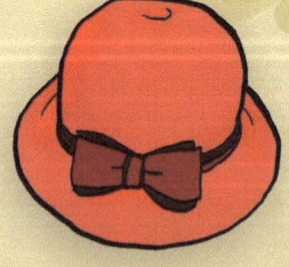

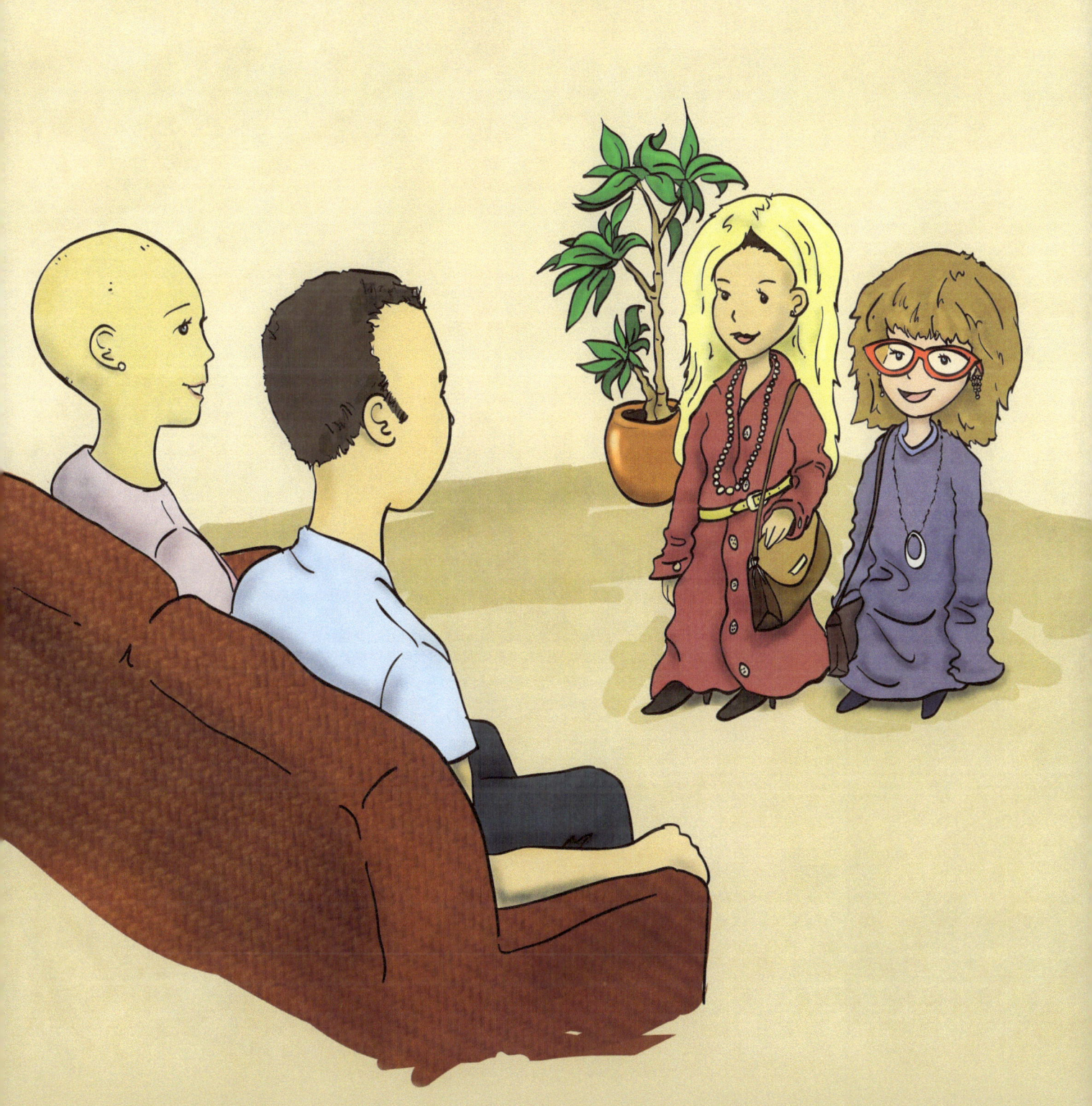

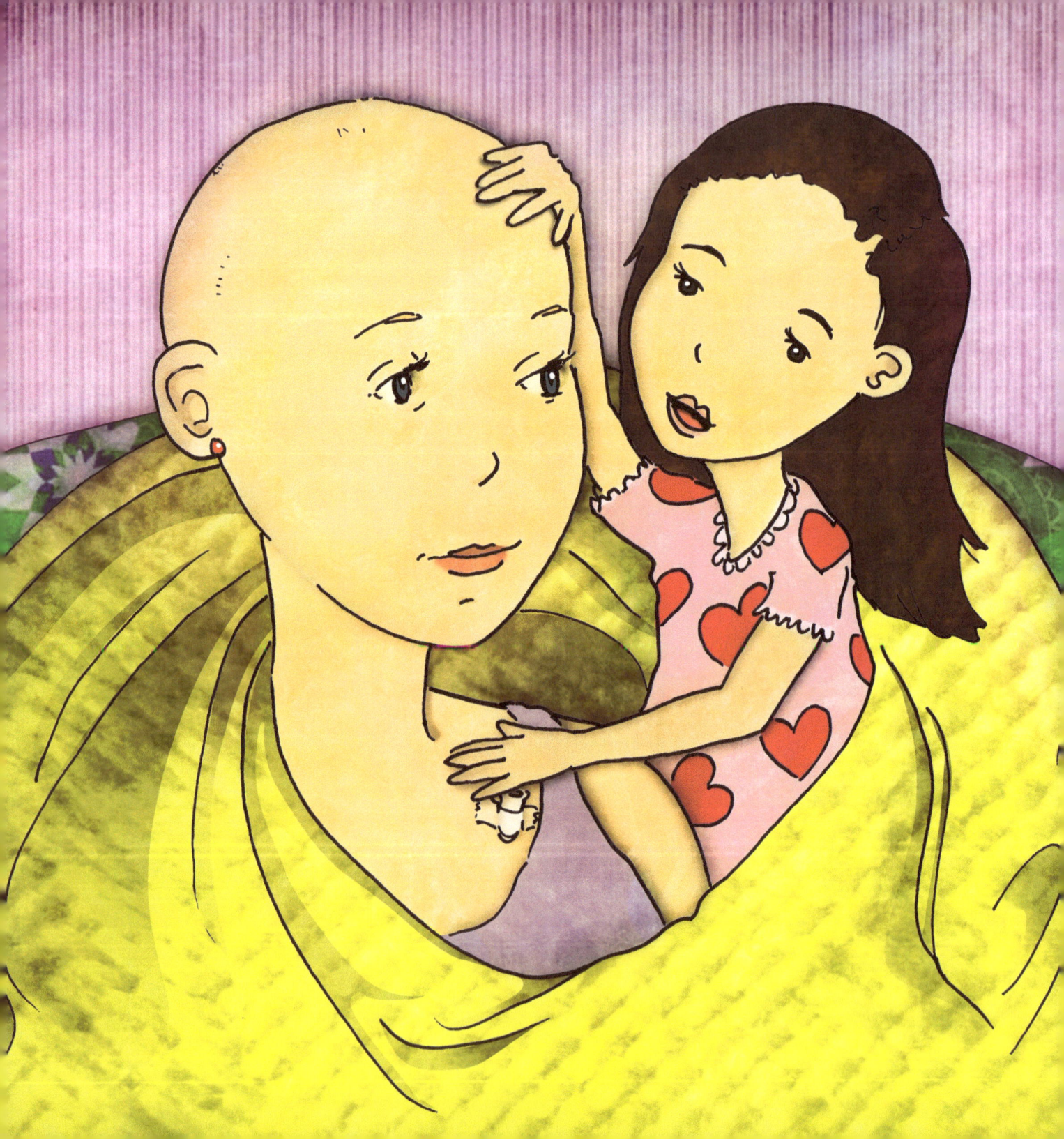

Sometimes I like to check and see if she's feeling alright.

I rub my hand across her head and then I hold her tight.

——————— ———————

Daddy helps us
every day with
all the things we do.

Playing games,
giving us our baths,
then off to bed with
a book, a kiss and
an 'I love you'!

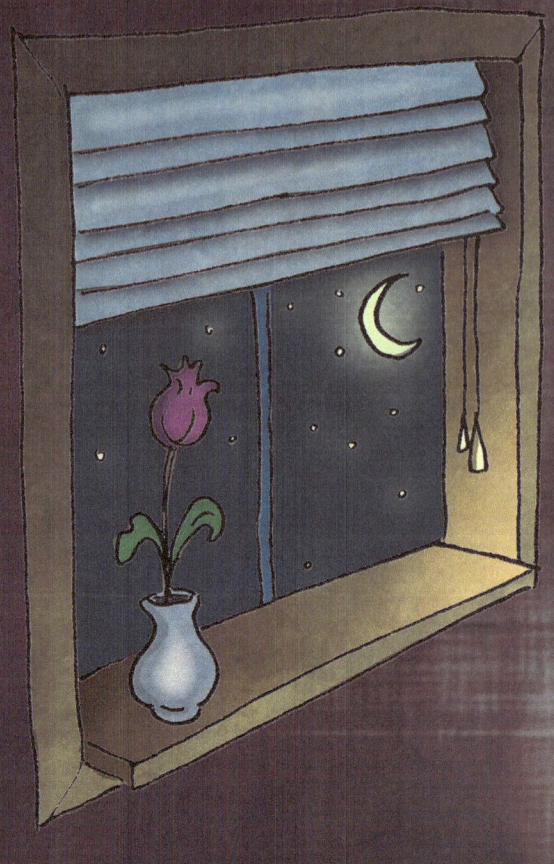

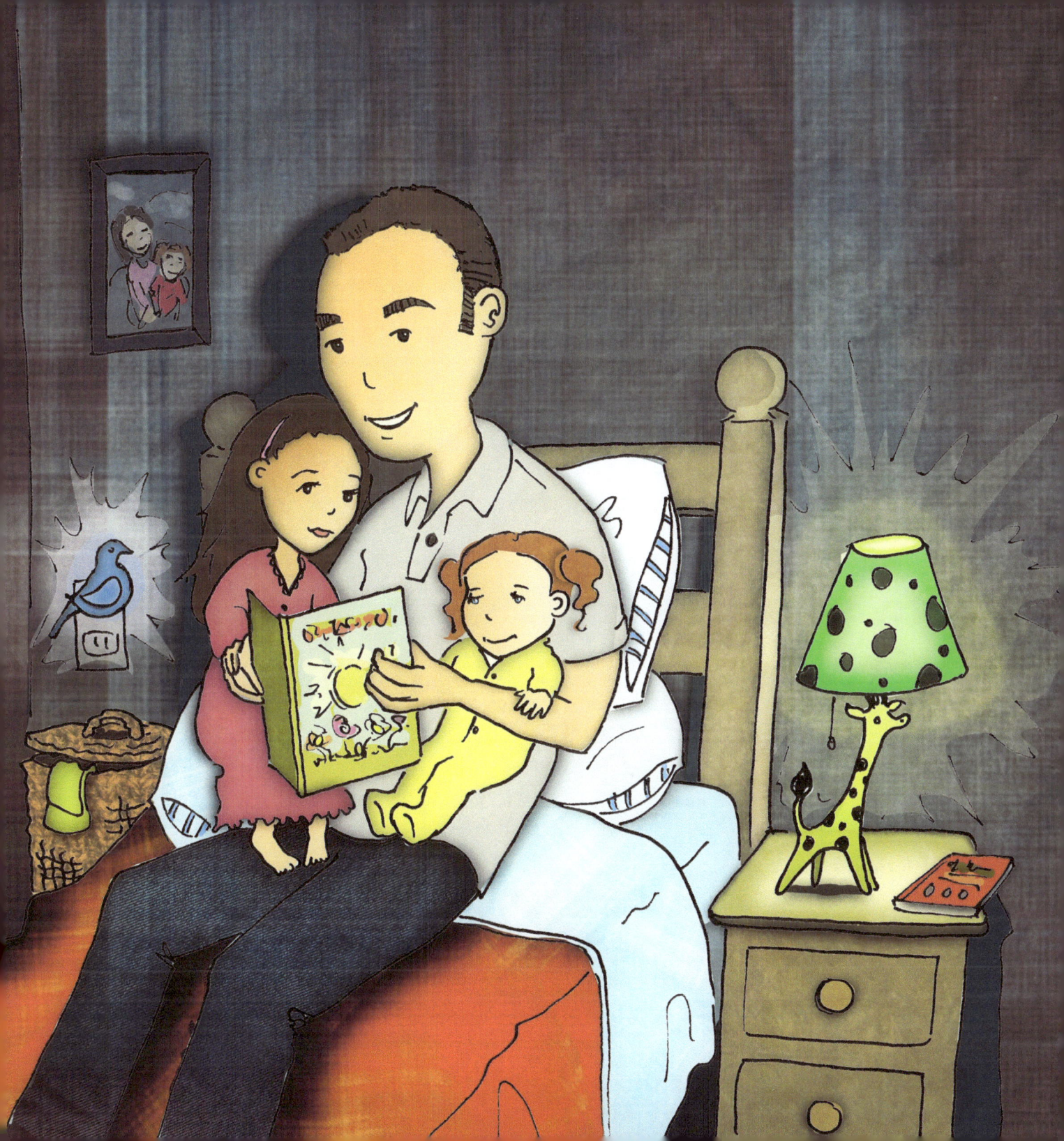

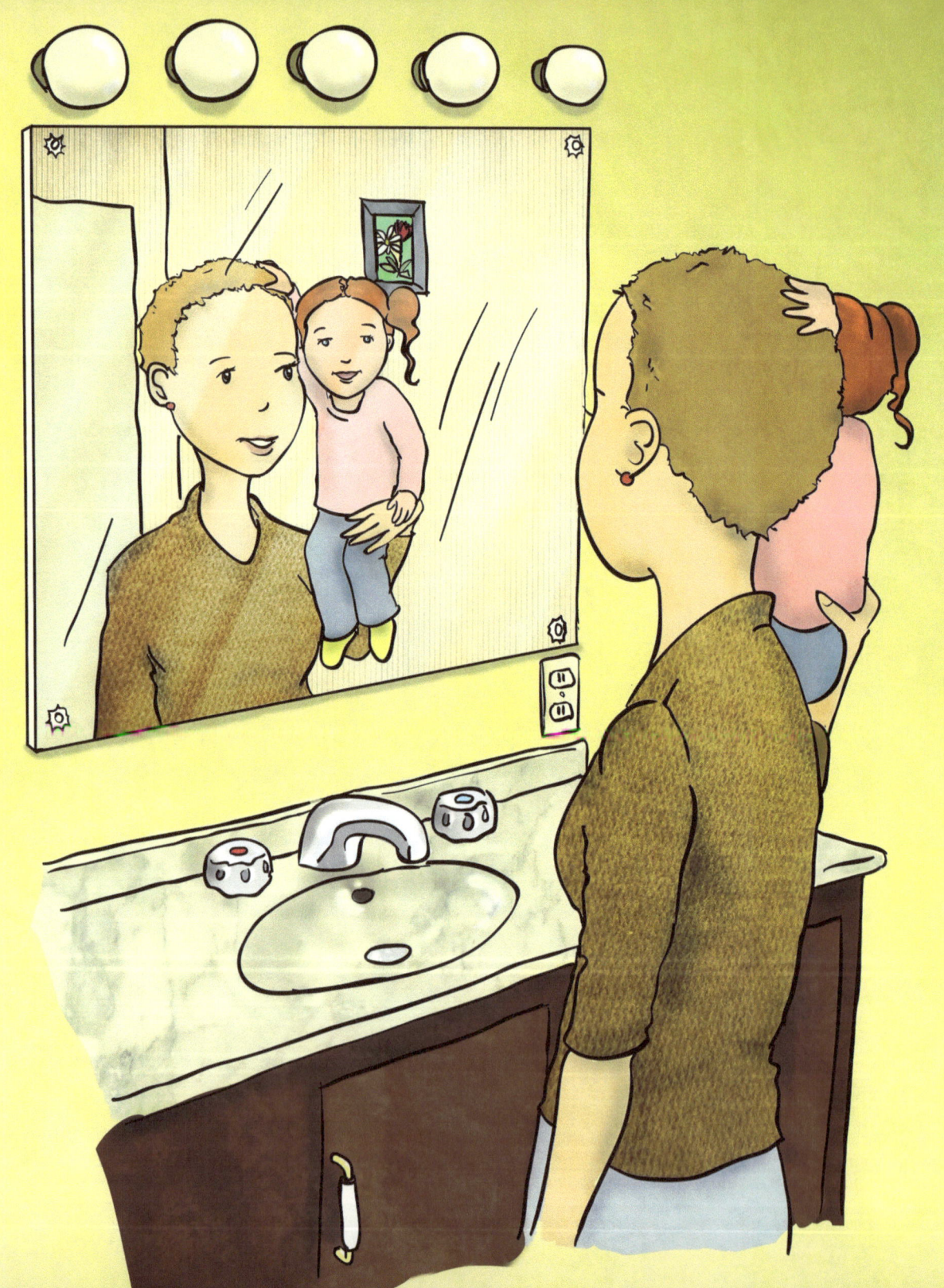

When Mom was done
with the medicine, her
hair started coming back.

We would meow and pet
the top of her head as
if she were a cat!

_____ _____

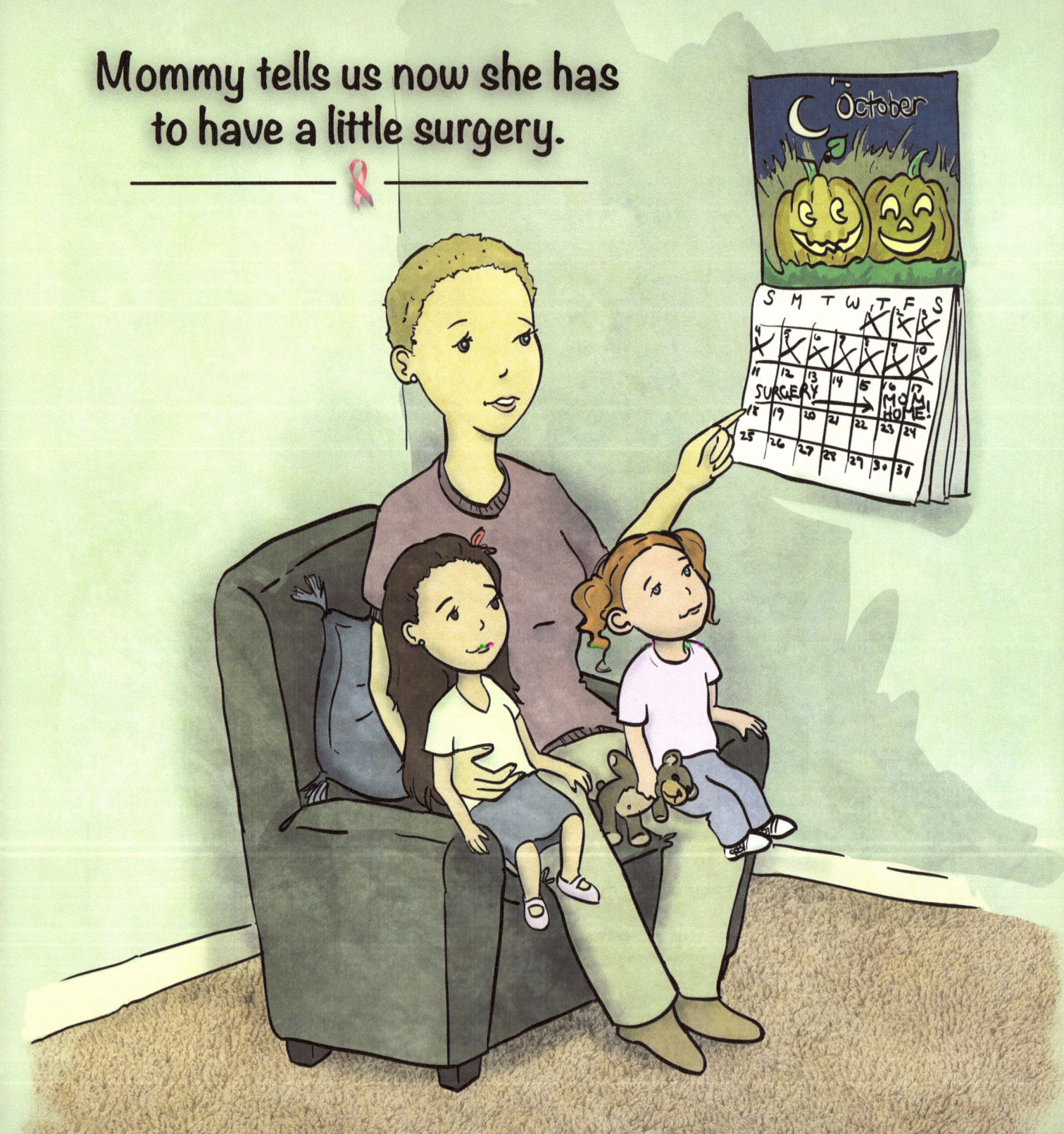

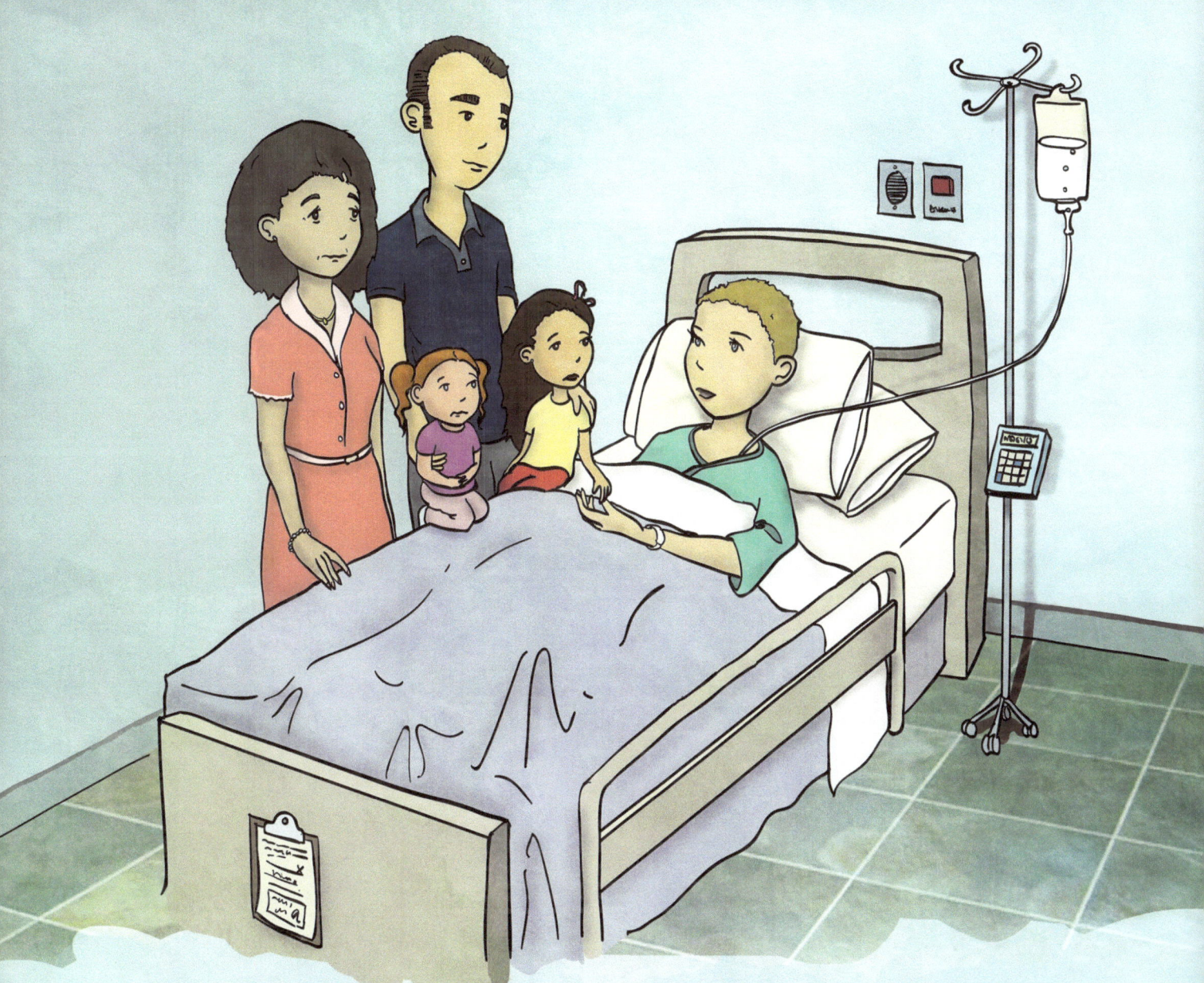

She says don't be scared and she won't be either, and tells us she loves us dearly.

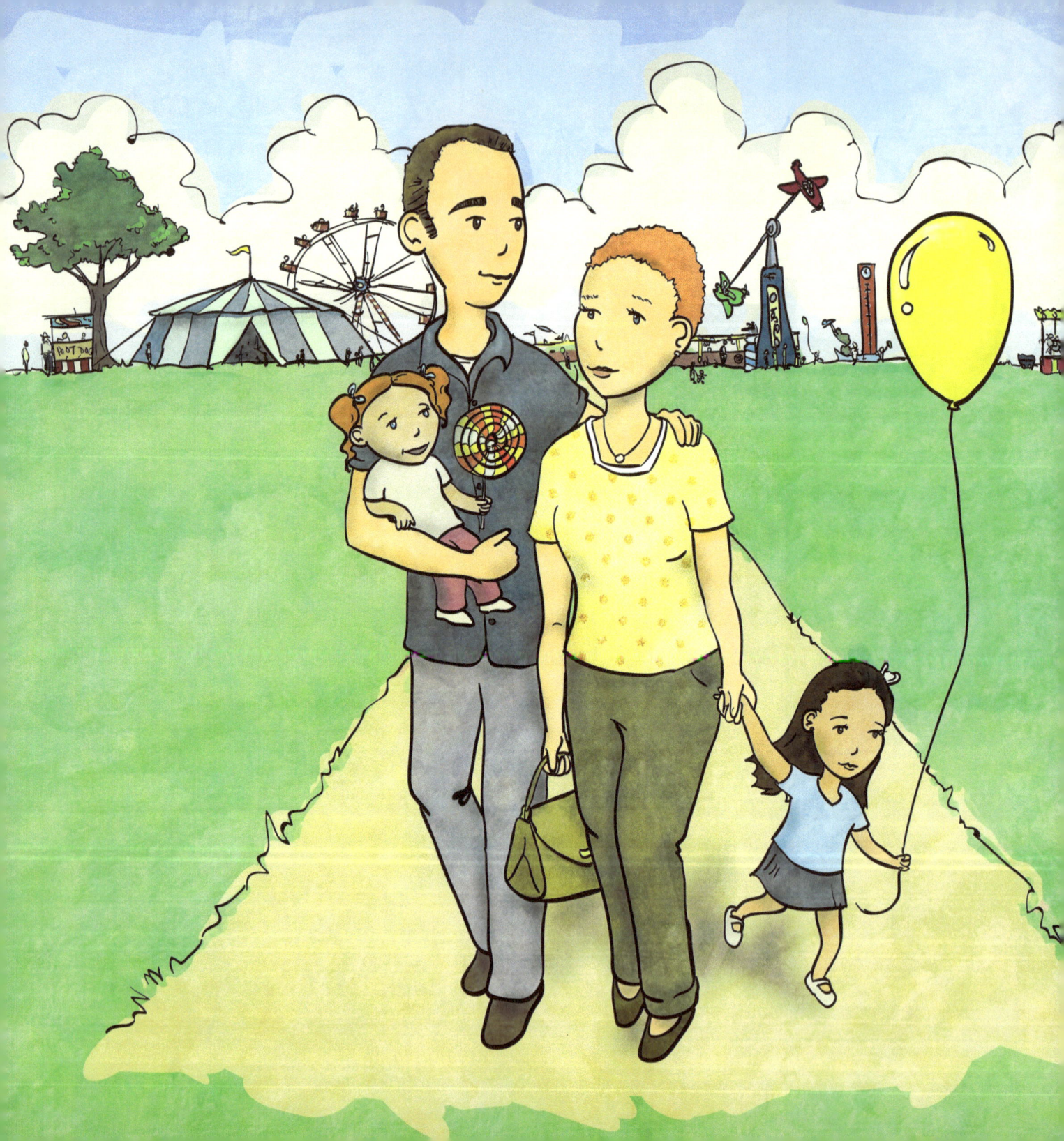

Now that Mommy is
getting better we do
so much more together,
and no matter
what cancer has done
to us, we never
stopped loving
each other.

——————— ⚮ ———————

I want to thank my loving husband Jayson who never left my side and always believed in this book.

My brother Joel for bringing my words to life through his incredible talent, you mean so much to me.

My family and friends for all of their continuous support.

And my doctors and nurses for giving the best care.

I have more blessings than I can count, and I love you all.